Wean that Kid!

Your Comprehensive Guide to Understanding and Mastering the Weaning Process

Kristi Patrice Carter, J.D.

ISBN 978-1517212506

ISBN 1517212502

For information, contact:

Thang Publishing Company

332 South Michigan Avenue

Suite 1032-T610

Chicago, IL 60604

800-441-9026

http://www.weaningthang.com

NOTE FROM THE AUTHOR

This book is based on personal experience, interviews with other mothers, and research conducted by the author and her freelance staff members. Although much effort was made to ensure all information in the book is factual and accurate, this book is sold with the understanding that the author assumes no responsibility for oversights, discrepancies, or inaccuracies. This book is not intended to replace medical, financial, legal, or other professional advice. Readers are reminded to use their own good judgment before applying any ideas presented in this book.

Acknowledgments

This book is dedicated to:

My loving husband Delanza Shun-tay Carter, for encouraging me to write this book, for being supportive about nursing our three children and patient throughout the weaning process, and for unwaveringly and lovingly playing with the kids so that I could complete this book.

My daughter Kristin Carter, and my sons Shaun Carter and Daniel Carter, for teaching me the wonders of motherhood, allowing me to share the joys of nursing, and helping me to overcome the challenges of weaning.

My mom Christina Tarr, who supported my nursing decision, assisted with the weaning process, and unselfishly came over as needed to watch the kids so that I could write this guide.

My father Lavon Tarr, for not complaining when mom came over.

I would also like to thank my researchers Geradina Tomacruz and Patricia Aaron; my editor Antigone; my graphic designer Alex, for designing my dynamic e-book cover; and my proofreaders Amy Shelby, Sasha Haines-Stiles and Jana Nickel, and a special thanks to Maree Blackston and Brian Bees for page layout and final proofing. Without your assistance, this book would not have been possible.

I would also like to give my heartfelt thanks to all the mothers and children who shared their stories with us. I am grateful for the time you took to answer our questionnaire, phone calls, and e-mails. Your stories, tips, and insights truly give this book special meaning.

Lastly, I want to thank my readers for purchasing this book and allowing me to assist you and your kid with this transitional phase.

Table of Contents

My Personal Story

Hello there. My name is Kristi Patrice Carter, and I absolutely love my three wonderful, beautiful, intelligent, and perfect children. Okay, okay, maybe they aren't perfect (heck, now that I think about it, they're far from it), but I do absolutely love them, from the tops of their heads to the bottoms of their feet. I love being their mom, and I know that because of them, I am a better, more giving and loving person. I also know that because of our nursing relationship, we have grown closer, and that bond will only continue to grow stronger and stronger. I guess you could say I created this book as a celebration of their nursing experience and a tribute to their weaning experience. It's also a tribute to all the other mothers out there struggling with the decision of whether or not to wean their kids, trying to figure out the so-called "right way" to wean their kids, and hoping they do the right thing. However, before we delve into those important subjects, I'd like to share my story with you.

I first witnessed the beauty and magic of nursing and the influence of nursing on the mother-baby bond when I was 18 years old. Although I had previously watched mothers interact with their children and had experience babysitting cousins and for clients, I had never babysat a newborn and had never even heard of (much less seen) anyone nursing her child. You see, nursing was never considered a big deal in my family. Formula was the drink of choice for all children—my grandmother, mother, aunts, and all my cousins assumed that "formula was just as good, if not better than, breast milk." I honestly never gave this subject much thought. All that changed for me one summer day when I accepted a babysitting position watching Jackie's newborn, Cora.

Jackie was a 30-year-old doctoral student who hired me to watch Cora while she attended school (part-time). We coordinated our school schedules so I could babysit when she had class and I didn't. On the very first day of this job, we were sitting around talking when the baby suddenly began to cry. Jackie immediately went over to the bassinet, picked up Cora, and pulled her close to her. The baby immediately stopped crying and instead started to make squirming motions, turning her head from side to side. Instinctively, Jackie lifted up her shirt, unbuttoned her nursing bra with her free hand, and cleverly helped the baby latch on. Little Cora calmed down, began making soft sounds, and soon drifted off to sleep. All the while, Jackie kept right on talking to me as if nothing were going on. At the time, I didn't know what or how to think. I guess you could say I was somewhat embarrassed but amazed by what I saw. I never realized a mother and baby could be so close or that the beautiful act of nursing could calm, soothe, nurture, and comfort a fussy baby. Jackie loved her daughter and Cora felt loved and loved her mom. While shyly watching Jackie and Cora interact, I immediately realized nursing is the most natural thing in the world.

At that "a-ha" moment, I must have been sitting there with my mouth wide open; Jackie started asking me questions about nursing—whether my mother breastfed or formula-fed me, how I felt about breastfeeding, and whether I knew anyone who breastfed. I confided in her that I was formula-fed and hadn't even known people nursed their children until just then. She placed the baby back in the bassinet and talked to me for hours about nursing: how it benefits both mother and baby; how it nurtures the mother-baby bond; how it provides the baby with nutrients, and so on. On that day, I decided I too would nurse my baby when I had one.

About ten years later, I married a wonderful and loving husband, became pregnant immediately, and vowed to form a close relationship with my child. I read every book I possibly could on becoming the perfect mother; I even decided I would have my child via natural childbirth. (What was I thinking? Just kidding, that was also a very positive experience!) I became even more committed to attachment parenting (nursing my child on demand, co-sleeping, wearing my baby in a sling, etc.). What I didn't know was how the nursing experience would ultimately change my life, how it would strengthen the bond between my daughter and

Wean that Kid! explores:

- Child-led weaning vs. mother-led weaning

- Are you really ready to wean your kid?

- Different weaning techniques mothers can use

- Special concerns you may have and what to do about them

- Developing a weaning support team

- When and how to wean your kid (a step-by-step action plan for you to follow)

- Activities you can do to enhance the maternal-kid bond during weaning

- FAQs about the weaning process

- 20 success stories from mothers and the methods they used

- Where to get nursing and weaning support

- Tools and proven tricks to make the weaning process easier

- Personal diary of a weaning mother

me, and how hard it would be to wean my daughter. I also didn't know the experience could be repeated for two sons as well. To make a long story short, the weaning process was harder on me than my daughter; as a result, she was relatively easy to wean. Although she nursed until she was 22 months (closet-nursed from 20-22 months—my husband and relatives still don't know about that), the weaning process occurred for us rather effortlessly; she was completely weaned before her second birthday. But every kid and every nursing relationship is different.

This brings me to the story about my oldest son Shaun. From the time he came out of the womb, he absolutely loved to nurse. In fact, at the hospital they called him "jabber baby" because he nursed so strenuously and frequently; as a result, my milk came in while I was still in the hospital. It came as no surprise to me that he was not the least bit interested in weaning at 24 months. In fact, it wasn't until he was 25 months that he was down to 10 nursing sessions a day. It wasn't until we hit the 27-month mark that we got down to one nighttime nursing session and one or two mini sessions during the night. And, by two-and-a-half, he was completely weaned. For us, it was a long, hard road to travel down the weaning highway. The weaning process took significantly longer and was a lot harder than it was for my daughter.

Then along came our youngest son Daniel, who shook things up a bit. Like his big sister and brother, he enjoyed the nursing process very much. He was a natural nurser from the time he was born and didn't show any interest in weaning at 17, 18, or 19 months. Then, at 20 months, he simply decided that he had had enough nursing and stopped cold turkey. He was done. No tears, no drama, no cajoling. He was done with nursing and that was that!

Although I have successfully weaned three children, I don't consider myself an expert on weaning. In fact, the more I compare my experiences to those of other moms, the more I realize that I have a lot to learn. However, I do understand very well how difficult weaning can be for mothers and children (especially toddlers), and so I wrote this book to assist other mothers. All mothers considering weaning need information, support, and knowledge about the various weaning methods available. Then, they can create an individually crafted plan to use with their special child. That's why I created this e-book, ***Wean that Kid!***, and **a website called** http://www.weaningthang.com, a comprehensive site to help parents with the nursing and weaning process.

So, without further delay, please sit back, relax, and allow your newly assigned weaning coach to help you and your beloved child get through the weaning process (assuming you're ready for this very rewarding and doable challenge)! I can't promise that your experience will be easy but I'll work with you to make it less stressful and frustrating for you and your little one.

Wean that Kid!

Let's Play Nursing and Weaning – Fact or Fiction!

B efore we discuss the various weaning methods, I would like to take some   time to share with you some interesting tidbits of information that we   found while researching nursing and the weaning process in general.

Let's play a little game: **Fact or Fiction?** It goes like this:

- Many cultures believe breastfeeding past infancy is beneficial.   For instance, Kung mothers in Africa breastfeed for up to six years. **Fact or Fiction?** (*Fact.*)

- Researchers have found that in most primate species, weaning occurs with the emergence of the first permanent molars; in humans, molars appear at seven years of age. **Fact or Fiction?** (*Fact.*)

- Research has shown that tandem nursing leads to competition among siblings. **Fact or Fiction?** (*Fiction.* Tandem nursing may build stronger bonds between siblings.)

- In a study conducted by Katherine Dettwyler, a professor at Texas A&M, 375 out of 1280 mothers who breastfed their babies past three years of age were still nursing their four-year-olds; 212 of those 1280 were still nursing their five-year-olds; and one woman nursed her child until he was nine years old. **Fact or Fiction?** (*Fact.*)

- Medical research has demonstrated that formula-fed youngsters have higher intelligence, better social 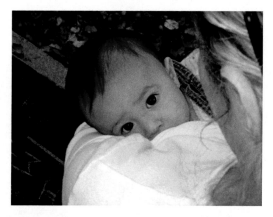 skills, stronger immune systems, fewer ear infections, and fewer allergies than breastfed peers do. **Fact or Fiction?** (*Fiction.* Medical research has demonstrated that breastfed youngsters have higher intelligence, better social skills, stronger immune systems, fewer ear infections, and fewer allergies than formula-fed peers do.)

- The American Academy of Pediatrics recommends a minimum of six months of nursing with a set goal of one

year or "as long thereafter as mother and child wish."
Fact or Fiction? (*Fact.*)

- Not allowing your child to wean himself is the absolute worst thing that you can do as a mother. You should only wean your child when they are ready (even if they're never ready). **Fact or Fiction?** (*Fiction.* There are child-led and mother-led techniques that you can employ. Both are appropriate depending on you, your child, and your breastfeeding situation. Using one method or another won't make you a better mom. It is up to you and your child to find the method that works for you both.)

- There are no valid reasons for weaning a child. **Fact or Fiction?** (*Fiction.* There are many valid reasons for weaning a child.)

- Deciding to wean your child will cause your child irreparable harm. **Fact or Fiction?** (*Fiction.* It is entirely up to you to decide what is best for you and your child. If you believe that it is time to wean your child, then it is.)

- You are selfish if you want to wean your child. **Fact or Fiction?** (*Fiction.* You are not selfish if you want to wean your child. In fact, you are extremely unselfish for attempting breastfeeding in the first place; that commitment alone demonstrates you love your child and want the best for them. Accolades to you!)

- Breastfeeding is the only way to show unconditional love to a child. **Fact or Fiction?** (*Fiction.* There are millions of ways to nurture a child and breastfeeding is only one of them.)

- Weaning is too hard and takes too much time. **Fact or Fiction?** (*Fiction.* Anyone can successfully wean their child with knowledge, guidance, and support—this book gives you all three!)

So how did you do? I got them all right, but then again, I'm the one who chose these questions based on my research! So, I had a bit of an advantage.

Okay, now that we've had some fun playing this game and learned some interesting breastfeeding and weaning tidbits, let's discuss the two main methods mothers use when weaning.

Child-Led Weaning vs. Mother-Led Weaning

What Is Child-Led Weaning?

The child-led weaning method usually occurs after the child is well over a year old. According to Katherine Dettwyler, Associate Professor of Anthropology and Nutrition at Texas A&M University and author of *Breastfeeding: Biocultural Perspectives*, "In societies where children are allowed to nurse 'as long as they want,' they usually self-wean, with no arguments or emotional trauma, between three and four years of age. The minimum predicted age for a natural age of weaning in humans is two-and-a-half years, with a maximum of seven years."

Also, children who self-wean typically acquire the majority of their nutrients from solids and often drink from a sippy cup. While self-weaning, they usually cut down on nursing very gradually (over a period of months, one session at a time). In most instances, they continue with only a nighttime, morning, or naptime nursing session (or a combination) for months before they are completely weaned. However, it is important to note this method is dependent upon the child's individuality and may or may not work for you.

Advantages of Child-Led Weaning

- Child-led weaning might be less stressful for the child and might intensify the maternal-child bond (if both partners are still interested in prolonged nursing).

- La Leche League International maintains child-led weaning allows for differences in children by letting them grow at their own rate.

- Advocates for child-led weaning argue self-weaned children are secure and independent.

- When a child is allowed to self-wean, he or she tends not to regress or want to resume nursing after it has ended.

- Since children seem to self-wean at a later age, they typically enjoy more health benefits than do the children of mothers who wean their children earlier. For instance, they have fewer food allergies from foods like rice and dairy.

- Mothers are better able to tame tantrums by allowing their babies to nurse.

- In case of illness, self-weaning children are less likely to dehydrate; when ill, children may resist food and drink, leading to complications. However, they are more likely to nurse when ill, avoiding dehydration.

Disadvantages of Child-Led Weaning

- The process may take a long time, depending on the child.

- Society looks unfavorably upon this method because children tend to nurse until older.

- A mother might feel embarrassed if an older child attempts to expose her breast in order to nurse in public.

- Opponents argue mothers do it for their own satisfaction and that it creates dependent children.

- It can be difficult to find people to support your extended breastfeeding decision.

- A mother/father may feel as if the child has too much control over the weaning process.

- Child-led weaning can be stressful for the mother if she is eager to wean and the child is not.

- After an extended time, women may not enjoy the contact and may even find it bothersome.

- Many women feel they have to "closet nurse" to avoid familial confrontation.

- Child-led weaning can cause marital strife if a husband wants his wife to wean their child and she allows the child to self-wean.

My son Jacob nursed continuously, day and night, for about four years. We co-slept, making night nursing much easier, but weaning harder. There were times I thought he was nursing simply for comfort, but as time went on, I realized Jacob was actually swallowing and eating, so naturally I assumed he was hungry. During the two-year period he was nursing, he would eat every two hours or so. I felt I should be happy to have a healthy and attached baby.

Sometimes, however, I stressed about Jacob weaning himself. At times, I was frustrated. Did I wish he would just wean? Of course! I have another son who recently turned seven, and I found it difficult to spend time with him because I needed to nurse so much. Nonetheless, I did manage to find time for both. For instance, when Jacob was sleeping, I always found time to do things with my older son. I even managed to tidy the house on occasion and do laundry.

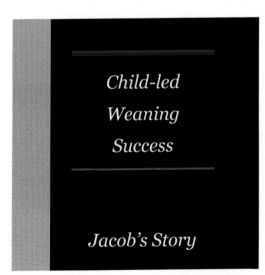

Child-led

Weaning

Success

Jacob's Story

Most of the people I knew stopped breastfeeding their children early. My child, on the other hand, seemed addicted to breastfeeding. One night, unexpectedly, he didn't nurse at all and slept through the night. From then on, he didn't need to nurse; he just wanted to cuddle. One day he even came to me, hugged me, and said, "I love you, Mommy, and I love your ba bas!" I nearly died laughing. He still didn't ask to nurse, but carried on his way.

To my surprise, not once did he ask to nurse again. I kept expecting it to happen, but it never did. He even stopped asking to nurse at naptime. Instead, he just curled up with me in bed. Keep in mind naptime was normally a time we nursed together. I even asked him if he wanted to nurse, but he just shrugged his little shoulders and instead requested we lie together. After the date he slept through the night, he never wanted to nurse again. In all, I actually found it hard not nursing, but I soon got over it when I realized weaning happens when the child is ready, even if the mother is not.

-Amelia Franklin, mother to Jacob, Chicago

What Is Mother-Led Weaning?

Mother-led weaning is just the opposite of child-led weaning. The mother decides it is time to end the weaning process. Although the child might be a willing (or unwilling) participant, the mother decides she is ready for the nursing relationship to end and takes action to wean her child. Here are some methods mothers might employ: don't offer, don't refuse; drop one feeding at a time; distraction or substitution; changing the nursing routine; or postponing or shortening nursing sessions.

Advantages of Mother-Led Weaning

- Mother feels more in control of the weaning process and can choose a method that benefits her and her child.

- Mother-led weaning may cause less depression in the mother because she has an active role in the weaning process.

- Mother-led weaning may cause less stress in relationships where the father is against extended breastfeeding.

- Metabolism slows during nursing. Therefore, women may be better able to lose "baby fat" due to a boost in metabolism after nursing ends (a big incentive for some moms).

- A mother who chooses this method may experience more support during the weaning process than a mother who allows her child to self-wean.

- Women are better able to control the weaning process.

- The fully weaned child might sleep through the night, benefitting both child and mother.

Disadvantages of Mother-Led Weaning

- The child may vehemently oppose weaning, causing the mother to question her decision or feel guilty.

- Depending on the technique, weaning may prove stressful for the child, mother, and other family members.

- Women may experience engorgement or acquire a breast infection if they attempt to wean too abruptly.

- The child may experience temper tantrums or crying episodes, or may feel depressed, sad or angry due to the mother-led weaning process.

My Personal Experience – Child-Led vs. Mother-Led

Although I initially reviewed the benefits of both methods (child-led and mother-led weaning), my daughter's weaning happened effortlessly, as we both seemed to lose interest around her second birthday. She became increasingly less interested in nursing and naturally dropped nursing sessions as she became older and more independent. Eventually, a day came when there just weren't any more sessions.

As for my son Daniel, he simply decided that he'd had enough and was ready to move on to a sippy cup like his older siblings. Without warning, Dan simply decided that enough was enough and stopped nursing one day and never went back. Although this method was easy for him, I experienced mastitis and had a painful breast abscess.

Weaning my son Shaun was an entirely different story. I knew child-led weaning would definitely not work for him—if it were up to him, I'd be nursing until he was in college. On a serious note, Shaun loved nursing so much and after a while, I became downright tired of it. By the age of 24 months, he was still nursing 20 times a day. Not only was this frustrating for me, but it was also somewhat embarrassing—especially when he attempted to nurse in public, tried to expose my breasts, or had temper tantrums because he wanted to nurse and nurse now. It also became problematic for my husband due to my decreased sex drive and his inability to handle the child's tantrums. In essence, my son's nursing was starting to cause serious marital discord in our family. Therefore, for the sake of my family harmony and sanity, I made a conscious decision to begin the weaning process when my son was 24 months old. How did I do it? The answer is that I employed a variety of techniques.

Different Mother-Led Weaning Techniques

You may be asking, "What type of techniques?" Well, I, and many other mothers choosing mother-led weaning, utilize the following techniques:

Abrupt Weaning Technique

With this technique, the mother decides to stop "cold turkey." She decides she no longer wants to nurse and stops nursing altogether. With this method, the child gets no real warning. The mother simply tells her child nursing is over; there is no more milk, and that is that. She then refuses to allow any nursing at all. The mother uses a variety of coping methods to ease the process.

Advantages/Disadvantages

When stopping weaning in an abrupt manner, the mother may experience uncomfortably full breasts, acquire a breast infection (mastitis), or even a breast abscess. Also, the sudden shift in hormones may cause the mother to feel depressed, especially if she was ambivalent about the abrupt weaning process or if the child vehemently opposes the abrupt weaning. This process may cause much stress for both mother and child, especially if they are unable to articulate their dissatisfaction with this method. Therefore, if you decide to utilize the abrupt weaning method, take measures to relieve any breast engorgement and keep a very close watch for any complications. Some warning signs include breast tenderness, pain, or swelling, persistent high fever or chills, and pus drainage from the infected breast. Any of these symptoms require prompt medical attention and should not be ignored!

Ways Mothers Abruptly Wean

If a mother chooses abrupt weaning, there are many tips she can use from other mothers. Here are some ways mothers "abruptly wean":

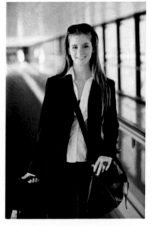

1. **Mother Leaves Town**

    The mother leaves town for about a week and separates herself from her child. She asks someone to watch and help with any anxiety the baby may feel while she's gone. Then, when she returns, she informs the child the milk is all gone and that the nursing partnership has ended.

2. Child Leaves Town

An alternative to the mother leaving town method is the child leaving town. In this instance, the child leaves the mom and upon her return home, the child is informed that her mother's breasts are now off-limits.

3. Cold Turkey + Making Breasts Undesirable

Some mothers go cold turkey and put something undesirable on their breasts (hot sauce, thumb-sucking deterrent, or band-aids) to make them less desirable to their child. They then use methods like distraction to eliminate nursing sessions.

4. Distraction

Some mothers use distraction during the abrupt weaning process. Whenever the child decides to nurse, tell them "nursing is no longer allowed" and give them something else.

5. Substitution

A substitution occurs when the mother persuades the child to accept something else instead of nursing. For instance, she may give the child a special toy or gift, a pacifier, or a sippy cup full of water or juice, or administer extra attention by distributing lots of hugs and affection—using any means necessary to distract the child when he or she desires to nurse.

I had no choice but to wean my son fast. For the first year of Ben's life, I took care of him during the day, and my husband worked outside the home full-time as a contractor. Then my husband was injured. I had to find a job quickly, or we weren't going to make our rent payment and those damn creditors would be calling. The good news was in two days, I found a job as an investigator. The bad news was training started right away and was in another state. I thought about not going, but we needed the money. Our savings were gone, and I felt we had no choice but to take this job. Looking back, I didn't have time to wean slowly. On Friday, I was a stay-at-home nursing mom, and on Monday, I was 500 miles away while my son and husband stayed home. It wasn't easy. While I was away for six weeks, I got sick with a breast infection, and my son cried for me every night at bedtime for three weeks because he always nursed to sleep. After the third week though, my son learned to fall asleep without nursing and stopped crying at bedtime. When I returned six weeks later, my milk had dried up and Ben was completely weaned.

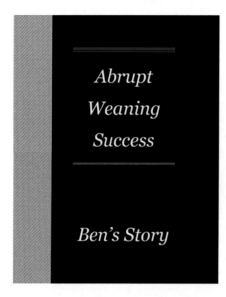

Abrupt

Weaning

Success

Ben's Story

— *Tracy Rhodes, Ohio*

Gradual Weaning Technique

In contrast, the gradual weaning method allows the mother to diminish over time the length and frequency of the nursing sessions until the child has completely weaned. With this method, the mother simply employs various coping mechanisms, which will be discussed later.

Advantages/Disadvantages

When weaning gradually, the mother tends not to experience full breasts, and the chance of a breast infection or abscess is lessened. The mother's body is better able to handle the shifts in hormones so that she may experience less depression. This method considers the child's feelings and allows him or her to better adjust to the weaning process.

Ways Mothers Gradually Wean

1. **Don't offer; don't refuse**

   Here, mothers don't offer the breast to the child but don't refuse the breast if the child requests it.

2. **Drop one feeding at a time**

   Mothers drop one feeding at a time until there are no more feedings.

3. Shorten nursing session

Mothers shorten the nursing session and then work toward eliminating the session altogether.

4. Distraction

If a child desires to nurse, mothers utilize toys and other distractions to postpone the nursing session, in hopes the child will forget about nursing.

5. Change in routine

Mothers change the child's routine, perhaps even taking the child on a trip, so the child's need to nurse decreases due to the new activity.

6. Postponing nursing sessions

With this method, mothers postpone the child's nursing request. For instance, the mother may say, "Not now, sweetie, later," "Let's play," or "How about some water?"

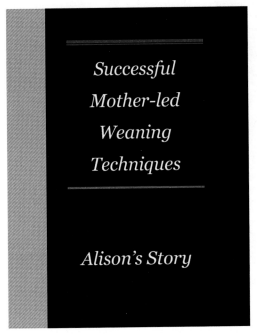

Successful
Mother-led
Weaning
Techniques

Alison's Story

I helped my daughter Alison wean at 33 months when her brother Sam was 4 months old. When I was pregnant, Alison nursed in the mornings, at naptime, and at bedtime. After Sam's birth, Alison's nursing sessions increased. She nursed excessively for about two months; tandem nursing turned out to be too hard for me, so I decided to speed up the weaning process for Alison. Initially, when Alison wanted to nurse, I took her to the park or used distraction. I offered her a special toy, video, or a special snack and read her a special book whenever she wanted to nurse.

After two weeks, we effortlessly eliminated her morning and naptime nursing sessions. About a month later, she began falling asleep after her daddy read her a book, so the bedtime nursing session was eliminated, too. After that, Alison began waking up a few times at night. Although tempted, I refused to nurse her back to sleep and simply rubbed her back and held her in my arms until she drifted back to sleep. Then she stopped waking up at night and then just stopped nursing altogether.

— *Amanda M., mother of two*

I never thought I would be able to nurse. So many things about the nursing experience terrified me. I didn't have the strength to watch extended tapes about the labor and delivery process, but I did take the time to read everything I could about nursing.

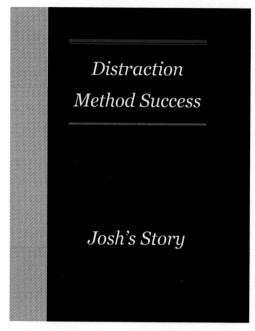

Distraction

Method Success

Josh's Story

For me, the idea of nursing a toddler was simply ridiculous. I remember thinking I would never be able to nurse Josh, especially as a toddler. I just couldn't figure out how anyone could get such a giant kid settled in their lap, much less nurse them. I used to laugh at the idea.

Then when I had my son and decided to give nursing a try, I was convinced I would never nurse my baby past the age of one. Well, as luck would have it, my little darling showed me otherwise. Josh proved me wrong many times, and nursing was just one of the many things he taught me about. Josh never hesitated to nurse after the age of one. In fact, he looked forward to it. He would hop right up, settle in, and drink up as often as he needed.

All the troubles I had imagined with nursing a toddler quickly vanished. I had no problem nursing Josh, finding a position for him to settle into (he took care of that), and keeping up my supply.

Sometimes I felt embarrassed by my lack of ability to wean him. My son wailed incessantly on the one or two fruitless occasions I attempted to protest. Occasionally I would catch an unusual glance or stare from someone, and in the back of my mind, I thought they might be commenting on my nursing an older child.

More often than not, though, I found people were encouraging. I was inspired by the number of mothers who shared similar stories with me.

Eventually one mom, who said she had nursed her son until he was three, suggested I attempt to turn Josh's attention toward a "lovee," a favorite stuffed animal that could "stand in" for mommy's boobies when the time was right.

At first, I thought the idea was ridiculous. However, I realized as time went on that the idea wasn't so bad after all. One day, I noticed Josh paying attention to a green stuffed dinosaur his nana brought over as a gift. It seemed for a spell to be his favorite toy-friend. Then I started grabbing "Green Bean" whenever the time came to nurse. I eventually started replacing one or two naptime pre-feeds with a cuddle session with Mr. Green Bean.

Eventually, I noticed Josh started calling for "Green Bean" at the most unusual times. Once we were in the grocery store, and I admit I was concerned because it was close to a feeding time. Josh looked at me, and for a minute I was positive he would cry out for his boobies. Instead, he simply threw out his arms and shouted, "Mr. Green Bean, Green Bean!"

Of course, at the time, the scene was a little strange, and I am sure that people thought my son wanted me to buy green beans. As it turns out, however, I think he was just learning to associate "Mr. Green Bean" with comfort and love in times of need.

I occasionally felt left out, and sometimes when Josh would cry out for "Mr. Green Bean," I attempted to offer my boobie. Usually though, he would just laugh, play with them a bit, and repeat, "Josh want Mr. Green Bean, Mommy!"

At some point, you realize your toddler is growing up and is ready to wean. I never thought I would nurse Josh as long as I did, but now I am glad I did. He is an awesome kid and we were able to wean gradually, without much trauma or regret.

I guess you never really know what to expect being a mother. I never expected to nurse, and when I did, I certainly didn't expect to nurse as long as we did. There were times I wondered if we'd ever wean, but eventually everything worked out for the best. I'm glad we did things the way we did. I'll always cherish the times we had together.

– Laura Zuckerman, mother of Josh, weaned at 2.5

I will never forget the day my daughter Kate was born. I was two weeks overdue and dying just to hold her in my arms. The day I went into labor, nursing her was the farthest thing from my mind. I just wanted her out!

The delivery went quite smoothly. I only pushed for 20 minutes, and Kate popped out with a beautiful head of thick, brown hair. I remember laughing when I saw it. Within 20 minutes after delivery, my natural mothering instincts kicked in, and I found myself bringing Kate to my chest to nurse. From that moment, we had a strong nursing relationship.

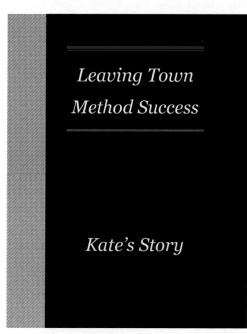

Leaving Town

Method Success

Kate's Story

Kate took right to breastfeeding. Amazingly, we never had any trouble with latch-on or sore nipples. She sucked so fervently, and I found myself with more than enough supply. I did pump occasionally, so every now and again, if something happened, we could give her a bottle full of breast milk. Most of the time, however, no matter what I was doing, I found myself adjusting my schedule to be sure I was available to nurse her.

I had never thought about extended breastfeeding. I figured most moms breastfed their newborns for about two years and then weaned, and that is what I planned to do.

Unexpectedly, I came down with a serious illness about 13 months into our breastfeeding relationship. I was sick and fatigued for weeks before doctors finally figured out I had developed a chronic immune disorder. To help alleviate my symptoms, I would have to go on medications that might pass through my breast milk.

At the time, I was disappointed and heartbroken. I was not prepared to wean so early. I also knew if I didn't wean, I couldn't take the medications I needed to start feeling better, and I needed to feel better to properly care for my darling Kate. So, after what I considered 13 very short months, I decided the time was right to start weaning Kate.

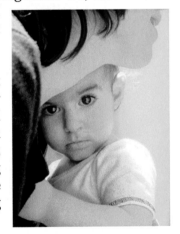

I knew about the dangers of abrupt weaning and did not intend to wean her immediately. Rather, I thought I could manage to wean over a two-month period that would bring us to about 15 months. My doctors agreed that as long as I took it easy it would be okay for me to wait two months before starting medications.

From everything I had read, I thought my best bet would be dropping one feeding at a time. I had so much milk stored from pumping; I decided to supplement one feeding a day with a bottle, which we had only used occasionally in the past. Kate didn't object too much.

Every week I attempted to substitute one nursing session with a bottle-feeding. Fortunately, Kate didn't protest too much. She had already been sleeping through the night for several months. Unfortunately, this process seemed to take a long time, and time was running out. That is when my mother decided to take Kate out of town for a few days to visit relatives. Since Kate enjoyed drinking a bottle, and I had plenty of stored milk, I agreed.

I was worried about them leaving, but Kate loves her grandmother, and my husband assured me being away could be a very good thing to speed the weaning process. To make a long story short, Kate had a great time and enjoyed having someone else fawn over her and give her a bottle. When she came back, she asked to nurse, but I told her "mum was all gone," and she was fine with that. She then asked me to give her some "coco milk" — chocolate milk in a bottle — and I did.

So at 14 months and three weeks, Kate weaned completely. Now, she is an independent little girl and enjoys drinking from a sippy cup. As a result of taking my medication, I am much better too.

I sometimes miss our nursing sessions, but deep down I know I made the decision that was best for both of us. I also feel confident I did everything possible to nurse my daughter and provide her with the best for as long as possible.

— *Karen Myrtle, Connecticut*

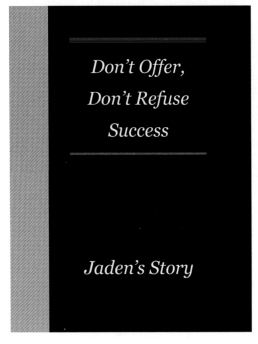

Don't Offer,

Don't Refuse

Success

Jaden's Story

Jaden was always a fanatical nurser. I called him my little barracuda. He dove right in as if every day was Thanksgiving Day. Never once did I have concerns he wasn't getting enough to eat.

I had planned to breastfeed for as long as possible. Therefore, it was no surprise to me when at the two-year mark I found myself still nursing Jaden. However, it was about this time my life started getting more complicated. I had planned to be home with Jaden until he was at least two, but now I found myself wanting to get back into the workforce. To ease the transition, I was only going to work part-time at first.

I know it's possible to continue breastfeeding and work, but I travel a lot for my job. Since Jaden was two years old, I decided the time was right to start weaning, so by the time I went returned to work full-time, he would be completely weaned.

Of course, once I had made this decision, I was saddened. I truly loved breastfeeding, and cherished every minute Jaden and I spent together. Still, I noticed signs he might be ready to wean. We had not had too much difficulty introducing a cup, and he didn't seem to mind using a cup for his lunchtime meal instead of nursing.

My plan of action was to go with the 'don't ask, don't offer' premise. So the first morning of my escapade, I waited to see what Jaden would do. We were into a well-established morning routine; right after he awoke, I changed his diaper as usual, but when we didn't immediately proceed to his favorite nursing chair, a look of worry crossed his face, and he said "nummy mommy, nummy!"

Well, of course, I couldn't resist, so I ended up breastfeeding. It seemed most of the day he was aware of his 'nummy' times.

Rather than force the issue, I gave in when he asked and instead ended the feeding a little earlier than normal. I would tickle his tummy and ask him if he wanted to play a game of hide-and-seek, or something of that sort. Much to my relief, he usually took the bait.

Eventually, I realized I would need to start completely cutting a feeding here and there. After a couple of months, I started with his least interesting, pre-naptime nummy. Instead, I quietly sat with Jaden in our rocking chair. We sang many songs and read books together. Much to my surprise, he happily went along, and within a few short days, we had eliminated that feeding.

Eliminating his other feedings took a little time. There were days when Jaden would whimper a bit, but it never got out of control. If he seemed extraordinarily upset, I would always pick him up and love on him for a good 15 minutes to make sure he felt secure and happy. My husband was a big help, always pitching in and ensuring Jaden felt loved and secure.

I suppose the whole weaning process took about six months. Maybe some people do it quicker, but for Jaden and me that seemed to be the right pace. I wouldn't have done it any faster. I still sometimes lament long-gone nursing days, but we have managed to find new ways to bond together. It's very exciting watching my fiercely independent toddler grow into a take-charge young man. I love watching him exceed my expectations every day. I always attribute his healthy outlook to our extended breastfeeding. I am glad things went the way they did.

— *Sharon Jamison, Michigan*

What Body Changes Should You Expect During the Weaning Process?

During the weaning process, various microbiological, biochemical, nutritional, immunological, and psychological adjustments occur between the mother and her child. For instance, in the mother, the composition of human milk adjusts to meet the needs of her child, so although the volume is decreasing, an appropriate level of nutrients remains present. Thus, immunological protection is not compromised.

In fact, "studies on the composition of human milk have shown when milk consumption falls below 400 milliliters per day, the level of sodium and other inorganic salts increase as the volume decreases. The fat, protein, and iron also increase while the calcium levels stay the same and zinc levels decrease. Milk produced during weaning also shows a decreasing concentration of lactose; fats increasingly replace lactose as the main source of calories. The calories provided by proteins remain stable. The concentration of immunological components is maintained during gradual weaning with a slight rise in the level of IgA, secreting IgA, lysozymes, and lactoferrin. Following abrupt weaning, however, the concentration of these components rises dramatically. Lipases (enzymes essential for the digestion of fats) decrease in activity during weaning, although bile salt-stimulated lipase does so only slowly."[1]

The mother, in turn, experiences several physical changes during and after weaning. During weaning, she experiences a decrease in her milk supply, and after weaning, her breasts may sag at first and seem a bit soft, but they will typically return to pre-pregnancy size after several menstrual cycles. If the mother experienced lactational amenorrhea, she will often become fertile again, and her hormonal state will change once prolactin returns to pre-reproductive levels.

---

[1] Brylin, Dunedin Highton. "Weaning as a Natural Process." Leaven Dec. 2000: 112-114.

I'd like to share with a funny story about weaning. I continued breastfeeding my daughter Sarah until the age of three. One day while breastfeeding, she kept pulling at my breast, seeming unhappy. Finally, she pulled away and looked up at me quizzically.

Then she grabbed my nipple, squished it between her little hands and said, "Boobie, you don't have any milk. Get me a drink of

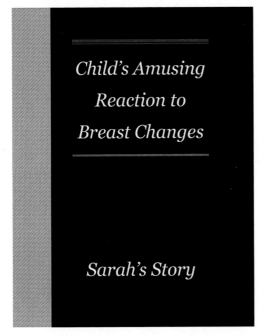

Child's Amusing Reaction to Breast Changes

Sarah's Story

juice!" I had to refrain from laughing and immediately ran into the kitchen to get Sarah some juice! The interesting thing is that I actually wasn't surprised that she preferred juice. After all, my milk supply had significantly diminished and Sarah never really seemed full after nursing. Plus, I was a bit tired of nursing anyway and wanted my breasts to return to their pre-pregnancy size.

From that day on, Sarah sometimes playfully tugged at my breasts, but she didn't seem interested in breastfeeding anymore. I never expected our final weaning days to go that smoothly, but looking back on it, I am thankful it did!

— Janet Smith, Kentucky

Wean that Kid!

When and How to Wean: A Step-by-Step Individualized Plan

By now you realize your child is unique – and so are you. No "one-size-fits-all" strategy will work for all babies and all moms. That's why it is important to develop an individualized plan to wean your child with minimal stress. By developing your unique strategy for weaning, you and your child will enjoy the weaning process.

Keep in mind that you should never feel forced to wean because other people find nursing (and nursing a toddler in particular) socially unacceptable. Perhaps you have decided to wean your child because you feel he or she needs more freedom. You might be expecting your milk supply to decrease, or you may have found it has already dropped off. You may simply have decided the time is right to wean.

You will successfully wean your child when you decide the time is right. Successful mothers realize the importance of paying attention to their instincts and their child's clues. Your body and your child will be able to tell you how the weaning process is going. Though this book will offer many tips regarding weaning, it is up to you to develop a strategy for personal success.

Getting Started

As a mom, you are the best judge of when the time is right to wean your child. It is impossible for an outsider or expert to determine the right time for a mother to wean her child. Deciding when to wean is a personal decision ideally based upon the needs of the mother and child.

Once they have decided to wean, most moms still struggle with starting, simply because they have not developed a plan of action. When the time is right to wean, there are several things you can do to start on the right foot.

First, sit down and plot out your plan of action. You don't need to develop a formal plan, but you should have an idea of how you are going to go about weaning. Gradual weaning usually requires slowly eliminating one feeding at a time, often at an interval of no less than three days apart. Deciding which feeding to eliminate is the first hurdle you will overcome while weaning. Take some time to consider which feeding would be best to eliminate first. If your child's favorite feeding is at the end of the day, you might consider, for example, eliminating a noon feeding first so the experience is not as traumatic.

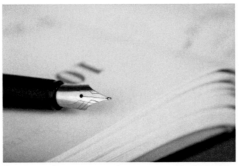

Many mothers feel stressed over the prospect of weaning. One of the best suggestions for reducing stress associated with weaning is gradually decreasing nursing sessions one by one. You can easily accomplish this by gradually reducing the time of your nursing sessions, rather than eliminating an entire nursing session cold turkey. If, for example, your child usually suckles for 20 minutes at a time, try allowing him or her to nurse for 15 minutes only. This process will reduce the "trauma" you may imagine your child experiencing at the prospect of weaning. Most babies hardly notice the slight time differential during feedings.

The change will be less noticeable to your child if you use a distraction to keep him or her from becoming aware of the decreased time spent nursing at the breast. There are many fun and easy ways to distract your kid, and we'll talk more about them a little later.

Keep in mind most children get into a routine. You have the ability to change this routine and thus make the weaning process easier. How you change your child's routine is also a critical step in the weaning process.

Start by changing the way you conclude your nursing session; if, for example, you normally cuddle and sit with your child after breastfeeding, try reading a book together or playing a game instead. This strategy will not only serve as an excellent distraction, but it will also keep your child entertained. You might also consider enlisting Dad's help after a feeding. Hand your child off to Dad and allow them to cuddle, play, tickle, and talk. Your child will be so excited to spend time with Dad, and far less likely to fuss at the slightly reduced feeding time.

Many children come to associate breastfeeding with love and affection. To minimize the distress of gradual weaning, be sure you offer additional cuddling and affection separate from breastfeeding. Consider allowing your child to sit in your lap more often; cuddle, rock, or read to him or her for a few extra minutes every day before naps. This one-on-one cuddling time will help ensure he or she continues to feel loved and reduce any anxiety that may surface because of weaning.

Another great way to alter your child's routine is to change the location in which you normally breastfeed. If you traditionally nurse in a rocker, for instance, try moving to the couch or kitchen. This will not only serve to distract your child but also help your child realize a new routine is developing.

Covering the breasts is another critical strategy all moms should keep in mind when weaning. The old saying "out of sight, out of mind" truly helps when weaning. You should keep your breasts covered when you are not nursing. Some children will want to nurse simply because they have seen your breast.

Another great tip for getting started is changing the order in which you feed your child. Most babies older than six months will be supplementing with some solid foods. Consider weaning during the time of day your child normally has a meal comprised of more than just breast milk. Feed your child first before offering the breast. Chances are he or she will fill up more on solid foods and therefore be less interested in nursing. You may even be able to eliminate nursing altogether during this time.

Getting started isn't as difficult as it sounds. With a little thought and planning, you will be able to develop a strategy that works well for both you and your child.

Visualize Success

One terrific strategy for weaning success is visualization. To succeed, you must first believe you have the power to effectively and successfully wean your child. If you believe you will fail, your chances of failing are greater. Time and again, studies suggest visualization is a powerful contributor to people's success in any endeavor.

So how exactly does one visualize successful weaning? Visualization can assist in various ways. The best time to visualize your success is during a stress-free moment when you have some quiet time. Consider spending five to ten minutes before bedtime visualizing your weaning goals and achievements.

You may find it helpful to write down your weaning goals. Consider at least two or three goals or affirmations and write them down.

Weaning Affirmations:

"I am confident my child will wean successfully without any emotional upset."

"I am a good mother and know what it takes to successfully wean my child."

Each night before bed, repeat one or two of these goals or affirmations to yourself aloud. Then close your eyes and take a few deep breaths. Picture your child eating independently and sipping milk from his cup.

Don't worry about feeling silly. Imagine interacting with your son or daughter in a pleasant and calm manner. Visualize your confidence and security, and that of your child. Visualize your toddler successfully weaned, growing, and developing into a more independent being. Imagine yourself jumping over the "hurdle" of breastfeeding.

At other times, you may find it helpful to imagine your life once you have successfully weaned your infant. This process will help you feel more confident about your decisions. Not only will you benefit, but also your child will benefit from your positive feelings and emotional well-being.

"Intuition as Your Guide"

Mothers know best when it comes to their children. By the time your infant transitions to toddler-hood, you will have a good sense of his or her personality, preferences, and moods. You will be able to tell if weaning is going well or if your toddler may need some extra time with you. Always trust your gut. If you feel uncomfortable during the weaning process, or if your toddler begins to act in an upsetting way, it is likely that the process is moving too swiftly, and you'll have to make adjustments.

If, on the other hand, you feel very comfortable with the weaning process, continue your journey. Don't heed the incessant advice of well-meaning friends and family members. More often than not, you'll find most people are willing to add their two cents, whether welcome or not. People are always willing to offer unsolicited advice on parenting issues, particularly on the subjects of breastfeeding and weaning. You are the best judge of your child's health and well-being, and you'll know if things are going well or need some adjustment.

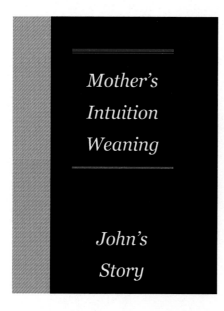

Mother's

Intuition

Weaning

John's

Story

As a first-time mother, I found myself breastfeeding long after my peers had stopped. When John and I reached the two-year mark, I realized I was no longer in the company of mothers who breastfed.

Three of my friends and I had found ourselves pregnant at about the same time. We were all due about a week apart from each other. I thought it was great that when John was born, he'd have three built-in playmates.

Naturally being of similar personalities, my friends and I all decided to breastfeed. I initially thought I would breastfeed my son for about one year or so. Most of my friends agreed. However, as their children reached the six-month mark and began taking solids, I noticed more and more they were substituting bottles more often than breastfeeding.

Most expressed much delight at the idea of finally weaning. My friends exerted a lot of pressure on me to wean, saying we could go out and live life up again, party the night on, so to speak. As time went by, I realized I was not the same person I used to be. I wasn't interested in "partying on." I was much more interested in making sure my son had the nourishment and loving embraces he needed to grow strong and secure.

While my friends gradually weaned their children by the one-year mark, I found myself alone in my desire to breastfeed. However, I did not succumb to their thinking. Instead, I continued nursing and felt pleased with my decision to do so. After all, he seemed happy and content and so was I.

About the same time most of my friends started weaning, I noticed their children coming down with frequent colds. John always seemed delightfully healthy, though, even though he was exposed to a cold or two on more than one occasion.

I resisted the urge to wean until John was about two years and six months because I thought he wasn't ready. It was about that time I decided I wanted another child. Right after I decided to wean, I became pregnant. As my pregnancy continued, though, John seemed less and less interested in breastfeeding.

At about the fourth month of my pregnancy, my supply started going down, and one day John looked up and stated, "Mommy's milk is almost gone, no more nurse-nurse. Juice." He didn't cry or anything; he seemed content with his sippy cup of juice, and that was that. He didn't ask to nurse anymore, and when the baby came, he wasn't interested in tandem nursing either and was perfectly content being mom's little helper.

I'm still friends with all my girlfriends. It's just I realized at some point it was okay for me to make the decision I thought was best for my son. I will never regret breastfeeding John as long as I did, nor waiting to wean him until we both felt the time was right.

— Janet Long, mother to Johm, Michigan

Tips for Gradually Transitioning into Weaning:

- Offer lots of extra cuddling during non-breastfeeding times.

- Spend extra one-on-one time with your child.

- Offer hugs and kisses when he or she seems upset.

- Distract your child whenever possible by spending time with him or her.

- Make time to focus on your toddler and coo over him or her like you did when he or she was a baby.

- Remind your toddler regularly that you love him or her.

- Gradually reduce the number of nursing sessions and the length of each session.

- Change your toddler's routine and offer distractions when doing so.

- Keep your breasts covered when not breastfeeding. Do not change in front of your toddler.

Monitoring Progress

Patience is truly a virtue when it comes to weaning. During the mother-led weaning process, there will be many chances for you to evaluate your progress and decide if you are moving too quickly or not quickly enough. Weaning can be traumatic if it happens abruptly and at a pace that doesn't match your child's needs. There are several signs you can look for to ensure your toddler is adjusting well to the weaning process.

Signs That Your Toddler Is Adjusting Well to the Weaning Process:

- Your child appears happy and content.

- There are few, if any, instances of mood swings.

- Your toddler does not cry excessively.

- Your toddler seems fine on his or her own and continues to behave in a normal manner.

- Your toddler takes an active interest in eating other foods and feeding him- or herself.

It is often necessary to supplement while you wean. If your child is under one year old, it may be necessary to provide formula in place of breast milk. Be sure to consult with your pediatrician before doing so. Older children can usually supplement with cows' milk, but some toddlers show signs of an allergic reaction and may need an alternative solution.

Your toddler should continue gaining weight and thriving throughout the weaning process. Most toddlers will begin eating solid foods in conjunction with the weaning process.

Monitor Progress Closely or Suffer Consequences

"A friend of mine thought weaning cold turkey was the way to go. Her grandmother told her she should just let her one-year-old daughter cry it out, and she would eat when she got hungry enough and not to give her any breast milk. For one day, the little girl refused to eat or drink, and she became weak. My friend took the child to the hospital, and they advised she was extremely dehydrated and warned her mother to take a more gradual weaning approach."

-Rebecca Carlson, Missouri

Are You Moving Too Fast or Too Slow?

As mentioned previously, it is crucial that weaning occurs at a pace that is neither too slow nor too fast. You'll have to take some time to gauge whether the weaning process is moving at an appropriate pace.

Signs Weaning Is Progressing Too Quickly

There are several clues your toddler will offer if the weaning process is going too swiftly. If this is the case, your toddler may show one or several of the following signs:

- Anxiety

- Increased crying or tantrums throughout the day for no apparent reason

- Aggressive behavior such as kicking or biting

- Refusal to eat

- Increased fear of separation or the dark

- Excessive thumb- or pacifier-sucking

- Excessive night waking

Mood swings are a common sign that weaning might be happening too quickly for your toddler. It is better for you and your toddler to slow the pace if any of the above symptoms persist.

Successful mother-led weaning is contingent in part on your ability to be flexible and patient with your toddler. Sometimes more time is needed. If you know this ahead of time, you are less likely to move too rapidly.

- If, on the other hand, your toddler is exhibiting no signs of distress, consider increasing supplemental feedings and eliminating additional nursing sessions. Your toddler may be ready to wean sooner than you expected. Many toddlers are fiercely independent and, in fact, have a strong urge to feed themselves and do their own thing.

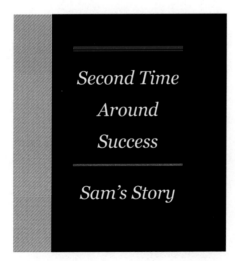

Second Time

Around

Success

Sam's Story

"I tried gradually weaning Sam when he was 21 months, but he would cry, fuss, hit his brother, and was downright hard to handle. It was just too stressful for all of us. I soon gave up and tried again at 30 months, and it was much easier the second time around."

— *Tina Monroe, mother to Sam, Nebraska*

Special Concerns of Weaning Mothers

Weaning affects not only your child but also your body. There are several concerns weaning mothers have regarding the weaning process.

Doctors and mothers alike recommend gradual weaning to reduce the impact of hormonal changes on a mother's body. Abrupt weaning can result in trauma to both mother and child. An excessive and sudden drop in hormones can lead to emotional distress and even depression for the mother. Gradual weaning will virtually eliminate this problem and ensure your body has adequate time to adapt to the weaning process.

Breast infections are a common occurrence in mothers who abruptly wean. Gradual weaning should reduce the likelihood of breast infections and allow your breasts to have adequate time to adjust. When you decide the time is right to wean, there are several issues or potential complications to bear in mind. They are as follows:

Breast Infections

Breast infections frequently occur in mothers who abruptly wean. The clinical term for a breast infection is mastitis. Signs a breast infection has occurred include the following:

- Localized tenderness

- Redness in a spot or spots on the breast

- Heat emanating from the breast

- Fever

- General malaise

- Nausea/vomiting

Breast infections are commonly caused by plugged ducts or cracks in the nipple that allow infectious substances to enter the mother's body. Plugged ducts can occur if your breasts are not allowed adequate time to adjust to the weaning process. One suggestion often given for treating a breast infection is continued nursing, which can help relieve the plugged duct. Mastitis may be a sign the weaning process is moving too swiftly, so reconsider your pace if you are prone to breast infections.

If it is critical that you wean as soon as possible, try pumping to relieve the plugged ducts causing the infection. This process will not decrease your supply, however, and will often prolong the weaning process. Your body must learn to reduce gradually the amount of milk it is producing. Most women who gradually wean don't typically experience breast infections during the weaning process.

Breast Abscess

A breast abscess is often the next step in the breast infection process. An abscess is a fluid-filled sac that forms in the breast because of an infection. It typically occurs when a recurrent duct in the breast is plugged and isn't able to effectively drain. It can be quite large, the size of a small kiwi. Although a breast abscess is usually more complicated to treat than a breast infection, and can sometimes require surgery, a breast abscess is relatively rare. An ultrasound can be used to detect an abscess.

Many times a physician will have to drain the abscess or aspirate it to relieve the problem. Most will recommend increased nursing of the affected breast to help reduce symptoms. An antibiotic is often prescribed to help fight infection.

Restrictive clothing and pressure to the breasts can also contribute to the likelihood a breast infection and subsequent abscess formation. A bra that is tight, for example, or anything that acts to bind the breasts can result in a severe infection.

Abrupt weaning is, of course, a common cause of mastitis leading to a breast abscess. On the other hand, the breasts have a remarkable ability to adjust to weaning without causing any problems. If you cut back on breastfeeding slowly and gradually, the chance you will experience plugged ducts and infection will be significantly reduced.

When Your Child Doesn't Cooperate

One of the most potentially challenging aspects of breastfeeding is working with your child when they are not willing to cooperate.

There are several reasons your child may not want to cooperate with your weaning strategies. It is possible your child may need a little more time. Some children are weaned more rapidly than others. If your child is throwing severe tantrums, not sleeping, or having abrupt mood swings, it might be in both your best interests to slow the weaning process to a crawl to ensure eventual success.

There are several ways to encourage your child to cooperate. First and foremost, encourage him or her to be independent. Applaud your child whenever possible, especially when he or she shows signs of independence, such as attempting to feed him- or herself. This will help your child feel more confident and interested in 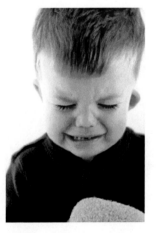 weaning. Be sure to exaggerate your pleasure and happiness when your child takes steps to wean and eat on his or her own.

Another strategy you might try is having another person introduce foods, whether solid or milk, to your child. This demonstration of praise will help distract her and divert attention to someone other than you.

Many children come to associate breastfeeding with love and find comfort in mom. It is often necessary to find a substitute "lovee," such as a stuffed animal or blanket, so there is something other than your breast to nuzzle up to in times of anxiety or stress. You might try picking out a favorite "lovee" together, and take the "lovee" with you when breastfeeding. Your child will begin to associate comfort and love with the "lovee" and not just your breasts.

Be sure your child is also getting enough to eat. Some children resist weaning because they are still hungry. Offer solids and supplemental milk or formula when necessary to ensure your child isn't resisting simply because he or she is hungry.

Remember, patience is also critical to any successful weaning adventure. If your child suspects you are upset or frustrated, he or she will likely cling to you even more and perhaps require even more breastfeeding sessions. If you show you are comfortable, it will help reduce anxiety and encourage weaning.

As much as possible, allow your child to feed him- or herself. Encourage mealtimes as family times. Have your son or daughter sit with you at the table when you eat. For example, show your toddler what a big girl she is by encouraging her to feed herself. Offer praise and affection when she participates and attempts to feed herself. Don't worry about the inevitable mess; finesse comes with time. You might want to allow your child to play with a spoon in order to figure out how to use it.

Never force-feed a child. As toddlers grow older, their appetites often decrease, and they might simply enjoy sitting at the table with you rather than eating. This still encourages healthy, independent habits that will aid in promoting the weaning process.

You and Your Child Aren't Ready, But Your Husband Is

Having a child often takes its toll on a marriage. Nursing mothers often spend more time with their infants than husbands and often, husbands feel neglected.

Many husbands want their wives to wean early. This can be due to a number of factors. Perhaps your husband feels jealousy over the intimate relationship you and your child share while breastfeeding. It is also possible your husband feels breastfeeding impacts your intimate relationship.

Regardless of your husband's reasoning, it is still important to remember you are the best judge of when you and your child are ready to wean. If your husband is ready before the both of you are, sit down with him and discuss his concerns. Find out why he wants you to wean before you feel you and your child are ready.

If you find that attention and jealousy are a problem, remember to shower your husband with affection as well. He may need to hear that you love him more often. Consider holding hands and sharing loving hugs and cuddles when the two of you are together. If your husband isn't already helping feed, he may be interested in introducing a supplemental bottle.

If intimacy is an issue, there are several ways you can express your feelings and sexuality without involving the breasts. There is, of course, nothing wrong with sexual intimacy during breastfeeding, but some couples or individuals are uncomfortable with the breasts at this time. This might be a good opportunity to try something new and creative in the bedroom.

No matter what the issue, you must talk with your husband and remind him of the importance of gradual weaning. Breastfeeding has many benefits for both child and mother. Ending the nursing relationship too early may cause unnecessary stress, not only for the child but also for the mother. If you feel forced to wean, you will drive an even bigger wedge between you and your husband. Chances are your husband simply needs to be reassured he is still a priority in your life and that you love him as much as the day you married him.

You Sleep With Your Kids

One of the biggest challenges mothers face is weaning while co-sleeping. Depending on how old your child is and how long you have been co-sleeping, weaning will probably take a great deal more time than if you were not sleeping together. Many consider co-sleeping beneficial for both mothers and their babies, but it may add to breast stimulation, stimulating the prolactin response and making weaning and decreased milk production more challenging for mothers.

Remember, too many simultaneous changes in a routine may further disrupt your child's temperament and cause excessive crying, tantrums, and mood swings. Consider moving your toddler to a big boy or girl bed before weaning, or wean and then move your toddler—don't try doing both at once.

For the most part, weaning will be much more successful if you move your child out of your bed first. Your child may associate co-sleeping with feeding whenever needed. If your youngster is still feeding at night, moving your child to a separate bed will encourage independence and reduce nighttime feedings.

That said, a large percentage of Americans allow their children to sleep with them routinely. There is nothing wrong with this;

it is a personal decision much like the decision to wean. Many parents in other countries sleep with their children as common practice.

Experts believe gradually weaning a child from their parents' bed is more easily accomplished between the ages of nine and 12 months. During this time, separation anxiety can set in and make it difficult for the child to stop breastfeeding. Often, successful weaning from co-sleeping occurs before weaning from breastfeeding. Some parents continue sleeping with their children well into their toddler years, however. The weaning process for these parents will be unique and gradual, depending on the length of time a child has been co-sleeping with parents.

As previously indicated, prolactin levels may also increase with a nursing child sleeping with her mom. Prolactin is the hormone responsible for producing breast milk. Children who co-sleep often touch their mothers more, particularly the breasts. Research suggests touch may stimulate the body to produce more prolactin. Prolactin production increases during the night. Thus, mothers who co-sleep with their children may have slightly more difficulty weaning than mothers who do not.

If you co-sleep with your child, you can still successfully wean, but the process will likely take longer. In this case, a gradual approach is best for weaning. Try weaning from co-sleeping first. Then, once your child is comfortable, you can gradually begin the process of weaning from breastfeeding. Alternatively, you may decide to wean from breastfeeding first and then wean from co-sleeping; too many changes at once will likely result in unnecessary distress for both you and your child.

Hi there! I thought I might share my story. My daughter Rachel is almost three and still nurses three times a day. I was finally able to help her wean from night nursing, and I thought our story would be beneficial to others.

Never once did I consider not breastfeeding. I never thought formula was bad but I preferred to breastfeed. I even bought formula and considered occasionally supplementing. Shortly after my daughter Rachel was born, however, I learned what I wanted was not necessarily going to mesh with what my child wanted. Rachel never once accepted a bottle. The idea of formula or anything other than breast milk seemed to repulse her.

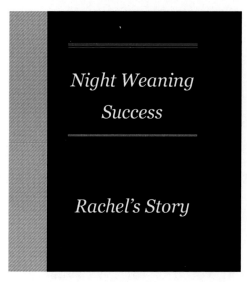

Night Weaning

Success

Rachel's Story

I nursed her discreetly anywhere and everywhere we went. Trust me, I wasn't the type person who thought I'd ever nurse in public. Yet, I found myself nursing her everywhere—restaurants, other people's homes, while shopping, you name it. Never once did anyone comment rudely and, to my surprise, many other moms offered encouragement.

I nursed Rachel without introducing solids until the age of seven months when she accepted some cereal. We also added some baby foods a couple months later. We co-sleep (another thing I thought I would never do!), and Rachel often woke to nurse several times during the night.

Lucky for me, just two weeks ago I successfully night-weaned Rachel with little difficulty and a lot of encouragement. I wanted to let others know about my experience, especially those moms who are frustrated at the thought of night nursing. I'm sure the idea a solid night's sleep might never come again is foremost in many night nursing moms' minds. I know I felt that way on more than one occasion.

I tried night-weaning several times before, but Rachel always cried incessantly, and I couldn't take it. I never gave up, and as Rachel grew older, I gently introduced the idea that "big girls don't need nighttime sips from Mommy, because mommies were tired just like babies and needed lots of sleep." I started by gently rubbing her back when she woke in the night or gently patting her bottom until she fell back asleep. The first night was the most difficult. She must have awakened at least 12 times, and each time she whimpered or cried a little, though she never fully wailed. She would always fall back asleep after a minute or two.

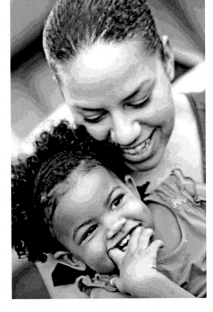

Take it from me, I NEVER thought she would be able to night-wean. I thought the ONLY way I would ever get any sleep was just to give in and let her nurse. Now, at almost three years, I have a child who sleeps beautifully through the night and doesn't need a bottle or breast to do it.

I wouldn't change the time we had together for anything. I truly believe our extended feedings benefited Rachel and me in more ways than one. I do miss the intimate times we shared at night. Looking back, the time we spent together nursing was very short. Trust me, you'll miss it. Take heart, however, and know eventually every child weans, and you actually may even miss the nighttime feedings and waking. Cherish every moment you have with your little darlings.

I don't see us fully weaning anytime soon—I'm plenty happy to have my sleep at night now, and I hope when Rachel fully weans it will be as painless as night-weaning because she will be ready!

I always thought it would never happen for us, but it did, and I am thankful. It will happen for you too—have a heart!

— Ellen, mom to Rachel, 34 months

101 Activities to Enhance the Maternal-Child Bond During the Weaning Process

One of the critical factors for weaning success is ensuring the emotional well-being and stability of your child while weaning. For many, breastfeeding establishes a close maternal-child bond. Weaning reduces the amount of time a mother and child spend together. Because of this, it is important to incorporate additional activities into your routine to promote bonding and affection while weaning. Below is a list of 101 activities you can do with your child to help reinforce the maternal-child bond during weaning.

Activities for children one to two years of age:

1. Make a big, soft, safe pile of cushions, pillows, comforters, and other soft bedding. Let your child roll around and jump in the pile.

2. Make finger puppets by cutting off the fingers of old pairs of gloves. Draw funny faces on them and put on a show for your child.

3. Make a sock puppet out of an old sock and put it on your child's hand so he or she can make it move.

4. Drape a sheet over a table or the backs of two chairs and make a tent. Camp out under the tent with your child.

5. Give your child a clean rag or dish towel and allow him or her to "clean" the floor.

6. Play peek-a-boo.

7. Read aloud, using big books with large pictures. It's never too early to start reading to and with your child!

8. Visit the grocery store together. Put your child in the shopping cart's child seat and let him or her feel, see, and smell the different items you are buying.

9. Have fun walking around backwards and sideways.

10. In the autumn, go outside and try to catch falling leaves.

11. In the winter, try to catch falling snowflakes.

12. In the spring or summer, blow bubbles with a bubble-wand and let your child try to catch them.

13. Play with building blocks. See how high you can build a structure before it tumbles down.

14. Take turns making funny noises.

15. Give your child a beach ball and sit opposite him or her on the floor. Hold out a large basket, such as a laundry basket or clean garbage can, and let your child try to throw the ball into the basket.

16. Shake a big sheet over your head like a parachute and let it fall on top of you both.

17. In the bathtub, give your child an empty can or bucket. Let him or her fill up the container and pour it out.

18. Take a nap with your child, or simply enjoy some quiet time in bed.

19. Sing a song to your young one.

20. Give your child a stuffed animal and ask him or her to "tuck it into bed."

For two- to three-year-olds

Every parent knows about the "terrible twos"—so named for the temper tantrums and physical exertions that characterize this age. Once children reach toddler-hood—at around two or three years—they are liable to become increasingly stubborn, self-aware, interested in others, and more talkative. At this stage of development, kids can perform more demanding physical tasks, such as climbing, rolling around on the ground, and jumping. Many children of this age also like to play with others and enjoy observing the world around them. This can make them a little harder to watch than a one-year-old, but it can also make playtime a lot more fun!

Activities for children two to three years of age:

21. Turn on the radio and move around to the music.

22. Visit the children's section of your local library for story time.

23. Play dress-up.

24. Put out paper and large crayons and have fun scribbling away!

25. Do large cardboard puzzles.

26. String large beads on thread or cord (supervise children carefully to make sure they don't swallow the beads!).

27. Play shadow puppets with a flashlight on a wall.

28. Go to the zoo.

29. When you get home from the zoo, make up a story with your child about one of the animals you saw.

30. Take a walk. On the way, point out interesting sights, animals, houses, clouds, or plants.

31. Go to the park and play on the swing set.

32. Go to a local art museum or gallery and have your child point out his or her favorite paintings or sculptures.

33. If you live near the seashore, pack a picnic lunch and eat it on the beach.

34. Give your child a piggyback ride.

35. Read a book together.

36. Make funny faces in a mirror. Get out a camera and take turns snapping pictures of each other.

37. Watch an educational program, such as *Sesame Street*, together.

38. Have a casual meal at a family restaurant.

39. Make musical instruments out of pots, pans, and spoons.

40. Buy or make some play dough (you can find lots of easy recipes on the web!) and let your child make shapes and then mush them up.

For three- to four-year-olds

From three to four years of age, children generally become increasingly graceful, articulate, friendly, and sensitive to others around them. Good ideas for children in this age group involve more physically demanding tasks and activities that aid the progress of language and social skills and help develop greater coordination.

Activities for children three to four years of age:

41. Ask your child to help you make breakfast. Make smiley-face pancakes by decorating them with chocolate chips or blueberries.

42. Skip down the hall or in the backyard.

43. Get out paper and crayons and draw portraits of each other and objects around the house.

44. Make up silly songs together.

45. Have your child help you with tasks around the house. For example, have him or her help you pick up toys and throw trash in the wastebasket.

46. Turn on the radio and have a dance contest.

47. Play make-believe. Pretend that you are at the beach or in a strange new forest.

48. Make a special trip to the library to get your child her library card.

49. Splash through puddles and mud together after a big rainstorm. Make a big mess of yourselves, and then come indoors, clean up, and sip hot cocoa or chocolate milk.

50. Buy some happy face and smiley stickers and place one on your kid several times a day.

51. Finger-paint.

52. Make paper airplanes and fly them around the house.

53. Go into the garden and smell the different kinds of flowers. Pick some flowers and bring them inside, and then have your child help you put them in a vase.

54. Collect rocks during a walk together and store them in a jar. Find a new and unique rock each time you go out on a walk.

55. Have your child help you make lunch. For example, make peanut butter and jelly sandwiches, and then cut them up into fun shapes using cookie cutters.

56. Set up a sprinkler in the backyard on a hot day and pretend the two of you are at the beach. Run through the sprinkler.

57. Make a collage with your child. Take some time to tear fun pictures out of newspapers and magazines, or use pictures from old holiday and birthday cards, and glue them together on a big poster.

58. Play hide-and-seek.

59. Pack a picnic basket and tent. Set up the tent in your backyard and have a picnic lunch with your child. Let your little one take a nap in the tent with you in the backyard.

60. Make a car for your child of a large box and pretend that you are going for a long drive.

For ages five and up

At the age of five and up, children are quite rambunctious and like to run around and play in an aggressive manner. They are increasingly verbal and tend to enjoy reciting nursery rhymes, speaking in singsong, and telling jokes. Good activities for this age set are ones that allow your child to expend some energy while continuing to develop good learning habits and social skills. They also allow you to spend quality time with your child even while teaching him or her how to be an independent thinker and doer.

Activities for children ages five and up:

61. Help your child clean her room.

62. Bake and decorate cookies or a cake together. Start by taking out your cookbook and reading the recipe together. Then have your child help you get the ingredients together.

63. Sign yourself and your child up for swimming classes, or just have a fun afternoon at the local pool.

64. Make a piñata and fill it with fun toys that are lying around the house.

65. Fill water balloons and store them in a bucket. Find a high location and do target practice.

66. Draw pictures on the driveway with large pieces of colored chalk.

67. Build a fort out of sofa cushions and pillows in your living room.

68. Make homemade ice cream.

69. Tell nursery rhymes.

70. Decorate the dining room chairs with toilet paper. Attach balloons to the chairs and have a special dinner.

71. Ask your child to help you with the gardening. Teach him or her the names of different plants.

72. Send your child on a scavenger hunt. Given him or her a list of things to find.

73. Sing into a karaoke machine to your child, and then have him or her sing to you.

74. Read a poem together, and then help your child memorize it and recite it back to you.

75. Make greeting, birthday, or holiday cards by cutting out magazine pictures with blunt-tipped scissors and pasting them onto folded sheets of construction

paper. Give your child markers to write on and decorate the cards.

76. Invite a friend over to play.

77. Play a game of chase.

78. Create a made-up language that only you two know.

79. Finish a puzzle, and then mount it in a frame and hang it in your child's room.

80. Tell a story to your child in a unique way. Consider using puppets. Spend part of your day making puppets together, then tell a story about how important your son or daughter is to you. Then ask him or her to make up a story just for you.

For children of any age

No matter how old your child is, spending time together is crucial to his or her emotional well-being. This quality time is especially true during the weaning process, when the gradual elimination of nursing sessions means that mom and child are spending less time together.

81. Set up play-dates with other children of a similar age.

82. Hug your child randomly throughout the day. Each time, say how much you love him or her.

83. Brush and play with your child's hair.

84. Hold hands while sitting, standing, or walking together.

85. Allow your child to sit in your lap while you are watching TV or listening to music on the radio.

86. Linger over bath time, spending extra time playing with your child in the bathtub.

87. Rock your child for a few minutes before naps or before bed and remind him or her of your love.

88. Enjoy a meal together without any other distractions.

89. Go outside, put a blanket on the ground, and lay on your backs, looking at clouds.

90. While you are doing laundry, give your child an age-appropriate task. For very young children, allow them to play with a sock, placing it on their hand like a puppet. For older children, ask them to help you sort clothes into piles.

91. Watch an age-appropriate movie together.

92. Make a set of "drums" out of cardboard boxes turned upside-down.

93. Get out a tape recorder and take turns recording each other's voices. Sing songs, make silly noises, talk to each other—just have fun!

94. Play a makeshift game of tug-of-war using a towel or a sheet.

95. Take an old box and turn it into a "treasure chest." Decorate it by drawing or painting on it or pasting pictures to it, and then fill it with costumes, toys, or whatever else you can think of!

96. Take a book outside and read together on the porch or the lawn.

97. Make and wear paper hats. Use newspaper, wrapping paper, or construction paper. If your child is old enough, encourage him or her to make "feathers" and other details out of extra pieces of paper.

98. Enlist your child's help in deciding what fun foods to pack for a picnic lunch. Then let your child help you pack the food in a basket or lunchbox.

99. Color in a coloring book. If your child is older, encourage him or her to make a unique, personal coloring book by drawing pictures with a black marker, then coloring in the pictures with crayons or colored markers.

100. Call grandma or grandpa and let your child talk on the phone.

101. There are hundreds more activities the two of you can do to strengthen the mother-child bond. Anything that encourages creativity, stimulates your child's imagination, and allows you to spend time together will help ease you and your little one through the weaning process.

FAQs Regarding the Weaning Process

Will Weaning Lessen My Child's Chances of Getting Contaminants That Have Been Found in Formula?

Human milk is the best first food for babies. Breast milk contains a variety of substances that are good for infants. Breast milk is natural and does not contain contaminants that will harm a child. However, there have been some rare instances of foodborne pathogens found in powdered formula (specifically Cronobacter sakazakii) that can cause meningitis, sepsis, or necrotizing enterocoliti (especially in infants with weakened immune systems). In contrast, in very, very rare circumstances, some newborns develop a condition called PKU, which makes them unable to breastfeed. Outside of this, there is virtually no reason you should wean your child merely for fear of contaminants in breast milk.

News reports often tend to be dramatic. A mother's milk does reflect what she eats. There are several things that a mother can do to reduce the burden on her body and its exposure to harmful chemicals and to ensure that the breast milk provided to her child is optimal. The consequences of artificial breast milk can be far more devastating than human milk. Human milk is a natural substance that changes in response to babies' nutritional requirements. It also contains antibodies that help a child's immune system fight infection. There is simply no other substance that is superior to human milk.

No matter how polluted the world is, breast milk is still the optimal choice for young children.

What Is the Best Method to Use While Weaning My Child?

It depends on you, your child, and your circumstances. However, the method that most mothers use during maternal-led weaning is the gradual reduction in breastfeeding method. They utilize this method to avoid physical complications like breast infections and abscesses and emotional issues like depression, tantrums, and unhappy children.

That said, by cutting back on the number of times you feed your child every single day, you should be able to wean successfully without too much difficulty. Just remember that the decision to wean is a personal one. Your child will pick up on emotions you are feeling. If you feel that the time is right to wean, your child will start recognizing your needs.

Are There Any Special Considerations for Younger Children?

Although this book focuses on older children, mothers should be aware that when weaning a baby less than a year old, you will likely need to supplement with a bottle (formula or breast milk). The best method for doing this is to begin by substituting a bottle during the child's least favorite feeding. Your baby will be more likely to accept a bottle during this feeding than during any others. You may express a little milk from your breasts each time you substitute a feeding, to relieve the pressure. Do not fully pump, however, because this will send a signal to your breasts to continue producing too much milk.

The best philosophy for weaning a child over one year of age is the "Don't offer, don't refuse" method. If your child doesn't request your breast, do not offer it to him or her. Alternatively, do offer the breast when the child requests it. You may start substituting a cup of formula, cow's milk, Pediasure, juice, or another approved liquid for your toddler's feeding while weaning.

Another tip for successful weaning is to feed your child solid food before offering your breast. This strategy will help fill your young one up and reduce the total amount of time spent at the breast. Eventually, you will be able to substitute a cup for your breast at the end of the feeding.

How Long Should I Breastfeed My Child?

Again, the decision of whether to breastfeed, and for how long, is a personal one. There is no right or wrong length of time for you to breastfeed your child. There are, however, some recommendations and guidelines you may wish to consider.

The American Academy of Pediatrics recommends that breastfeeding continue for a minimum of 12 months. After this, the breastfeeding relationship can be continued for as long as desired. In many European countries, children are breastfed for two years or more. In the United States, it is much less common and often considered taboo for women to breastfeed their children much later than two years. There is no right or wrong answer, however.

You can decide when the time is right to wean your child. Remember that as a child gets older, their nutritional needs will change. Most children typically receive solid foods around six months old. Most doctors recommend that you attempt to breastfeed your child for a minimum of six months to ensure that your child gets as many benefits as possible from breastfeeding. Most babies will breastfeed for much longer than this, though, particularly if you do not have a desire to begin the weaning process.

I'm Pregnant and Still Nursing My Toddler—Must I Wean Now?

Even many doctors are under the mistaken impression that once a woman gets pregnant, she has to wean. By and large, most women can continue breastfeeding their toddler even after they get pregnant. Many mothers, in fact, continue to breastfeed their toddlers for the duration of their pregnancies.

Many friends and family members, and even physicians, might express concerns that breastfeeding while pregnant will compromise the health of your unborn baby. There is no evidence to support this fear, however. Uterine contractions are a concern for other mothers. It is true that uterine contractions are experienced during breastfeeding, but uterine contractions also occur as a normal part of pregnancy. They may result from sexual activity and even exercise. These contractions are not believed to be harmful to your baby early in pregnancy. In circumstances where a mother has a high-risk pregnancy, it is a good idea to consult with a specialist to determine whether to continue breastfeeding.

Most women who decide to breastfeed during pregnancy will need extra rest. Breastfeeding in and of itself requires extra energy. Multiply that by two if you are pregnant. Consider napping when your toddler naps to get some extra rest during the day.

Another common problem pregnant mothers have while breastfeeding is tender nipples. Altering your child's position at the breast may help alleviate some of the tenderness. Usually this tenderness is short-lived, lasting only for a brief time at the beginning of a feeding. If your child is older, you may encourage him or her to nurse gently to help alleviate some of the discomfort.

Pregnant mothers who are breastfeeding may find that their milk supply drops off or decreases slightly at or around the fourth month of pregnancy. For babies less than one year old, supplementation is often needed to ensure adequate weight gain. This supplementation may not be the case with an older toddler. Increasing the number of nursing sessions may help alleviate this problem.

Some babies naturally wean when their mothers are pregnant. Pregnancy often changes the flavor of breast milk, and some toddlers find this change distasteful. Others happily nurse without seeming to notice the change.

If you do decide that it is best to wean your toddler while pregnant, the best method is to do so gradually. Try substituting one feeding at a time during the day, and change up your toddler's routine. Remember that extra love and affection will help ease the transition to weaning.

After your new baby is born, it is possible that your weaned toddler will take a renewed interest in breastfeeding. In many cases, your toddler is simply curious and wants to taste the breast milk. Many will not remember how to suckle, whereas others may find the taste unappealing. Still others are more than happy to start breastfeeding again. If you have weaned your toddler and are not interested in breastfeeding them again, you should offer them a taste with a cup or a spoon.

Nursing an infant and a toddler together is referred to as tandem nursing.

My Child Has Weaned Before I Was Ready. Help!

Weaning can be emotionally taxing, not only for children but also for mothers. Many hormones in the mother's body change when breastfeeding stops. Some mothers feel rejected when their toddler no longer desires to breastfeed. There are many different reasons why a toddler decides to wean early. A child who is used to frequent bottle-feedings or pacifiers, for example, may lose interest in the breast or find the process of breastfeeding too time-consuming.

Older toddlers are actively interested in eating more solid foods, and so their tendency to breastfeed naturally diminishes.

Remember, however, that weaning is a natural process. Your baby may simply be independent-minded and ready to move on.

If you are pregnant, your baby may simply no longer enjoy the taste of your breast milk. Revel in your child's growth, and enjoy the new experiences and challenges the two of you will face in the coming years.

My Baby Is Suddenly Refusing to Breastfeed. Does That Mean It's Time to Wean?

There are many different reasons why your baby may suddenly seem disinterested in breastfeeding. These temporary "strikes" may come about in a variety of ways.

Most babies who are truly ready to wean still do so gradually rather than abruptly. It is, therefore, more likely that something else is going on. Among some of the more common reasons that your baby might temporarily refuse to nurse are the following:

- A sudden change in your routine

- A move to a new house or environment

- The introduction of a new family member or baby

- Injury or illness that causes discomfort

- Teething—this is a common cause of a temporary nursing strike, and usually goes away in a couple of days

- A change in mother's health

- A change in hygiene habits, such as the use of a new soap or perfume that may confuse baby

- A change in your behavior

If your baby is teething, you can try offering teething rings or cold and damp washcloths to help alleviate pain or discomfort. If you want your baby to return to the breast as soon as possible, you should be persistent yet patient. If an illness is to blame, cuddle and hold your baby as much as possible, encouraging but not forcing her to take your breast.

During a strike, it will probably be necessary for you to pump to reduce engorgement of your breasts. Reducing stimulation might also help re-encourage a baby to begin nursing again.

If you are ready to wean, you might consider this a good time to start gradually reducing feedings. Your baby might be ready to start feeding more independently, but still gradually. Try never to stop feeding all at once, as this can have ill effects for both you and your baby.

My Doctor Says I Must Wean for Medical Reasons. What Should I Do?

Many doctors mistakenly believe that weaning must occur under conditions that do not always warrant it. Pregnancy is a good example. Your physician might recommend weaning if you need to take a medication that will get into the breast milk and potentially cause harm to your child. It may be possible to wean partially or temporarily.

The decision to wean will ultimately be yours. Depending on the age of your child, you may need to supplement with formula. You should still attempt to wean gradually to reduce the chance of infection and discomfort. Consider researching the reason for weaning on your own and getting a second opinion before you decide whether you are ready to wean yet or not.

Will Weaning Make My Life Better?

If you feel that you might be ready to wean, you should consider the weaning process to decide if it will make your life better. If you are in the early weeks of breastfeeding and find breastfeeding uncomfortable, you may find that things get easier if you stick it out for another week or two. If you are experiencing discomfort, there may be techniques you can try to reposition your child to improve your breastfeeding relationship. Most physicians recommend breastfeeding for the first year of a baby's life.

That said, if you are looking to gain some independence and feel that your child is old enough to wean, weaning may be the right decision for you. With weaning come many new challenges, including addressing a child's newfound independence. Some mothers feel that they will have less pressure from others if they wean. No matter what your circumstance is, people are likely to continue offering unsolicited advice whenever they feel the time is right.

Weaning comes with many other responsibilities. If you wean a baby who is less than one-year-old, you'll need to supplement with bottles, and the bottles will need to be regularly cleaned. You will also need to pay more attention to your baby and offer alternative forms of affection and interaction to foster the maternal-kid bond. Some babies struggle with weaning and may go through a period of mood swings and difficulty sleeping.

By weaning, you trade one relationship with your child for another. Weaning may or may not make your life easier, depending on your outlook. Remember that with each new developmental milestone in a baby's life come new challenges and new rewards. If you feel that the time is right to wean, then there is no reason you shouldn't begin the gradual process.

How Do I Handle Criticism About Breastfeeding?

Remarkably, people always seem to find time to share their opinions and attitudes about a mother's choices, whether solicited or not. Breastfeeding is often a hot topic for criticism and debate. There are many things you can do to respond to criticism about breastfeeding.

First, consider addressing the criticism directly. Ask the person who is criticizing you if he or she wouldn't mind talking with you about something important, and then let him or her know how the criticism makes you feel. Avoid accusatory sentences starting with "You" and instead focus on your feelings and statements that begin with "I."

Consider sharing with critics the benefits of breastfeeding. Quote your doctor and the numerous studies that support extended breastfeeding as best for child and mother.

Remind your critics that breastfeeding is an individual decision. Let them know you care about them and their opinions, but also inform them that you have fully researched the matter and are positive that you are doing what is best for your child.

Let them know how much criticism does not appeal to you, and that it makes you feel sad, upset, and angry.

It never hurts to thank people for their advice. You don't have to heed it or even consider it, however; just casually smile and change the subject, or simply walk away.

Tell your critics you appreciate their concern for your child, then change the subject.

Tips for Avoiding Criticism:

- If at all possible, enjoy your breastfeeding sessions discreetly. If you don't mind showing them to the world, then you probably don't have an issue with criticism.

- Do not allow a discussion to continue if you feel it is going the wrong way. Change the subject or excuse yourself for the time being.

- Assure the person offering advice that you respect his or her opinion, but also assure them that you have made the decision for you and your child. Let them know you are not interested in discussing the issue further.

- Focus on topics that you have in common, rather than on subjects where you might have differing opinions, such as child-rearing philosophies.

Remember that no matter the stage of life your child is in, people will always find an excuse to contribute their opinions, whether welcome or not. Rise above other people's insecurities and criticisms and have confidence—you truly know what is best for your child. Consider the possibility that the naysayers are typically uncertain about their child-rearing strategies, and that this insecurity might be fueling the fire of their criticism.

You can always prepare yourself in advance for a potential onslaught. That way you are never caught off-guard when criticism rears its ugly head.

What Is the Father's Role in the Breastfeeding Relationship/Weaning Process?

It is very important that children have a strong relationship with both mother and father. Younger children especially need constant physical contact. Whether children are still breastfeeding or have begun weaning, fathers play a critical role in their development. It is important for children to spend time cuddling and getting to know both parents.

A father can help feed the child by occasionally offering a bottle. While breastfeeding, a father can often cuddle and hold a child just after breastfeeding, when the child is content and wants nothing more than companionship.

During the weaning process, a father's presence is critical. Remember that children who are being weaned need more cuddle time than ever and require lots of attention and affection to be showered on them. Fathers can help by taking time out of their day to interact with their children, playing games, talking and reading books together, and so on. A father can also help out by introducing solid foods and milk cups to a weaning child so that the child comes to associate love and affection and a new routine with both father and mother.

Which Nursing Sessions Should I Drop As My Baby Gets Older?

It's really up to you as to which nursing session you drop next. Many moms drop the least favorite session first and then proceed to drop others. For instance, if your toddler obtains the majority of her nutrients from lunch and prefers to fall asleep being rocked, you may consider dropping the lunchtime nursing session first. It's up to you and your baby.

Do I Give Him Cow's Milk AT ALL While I'm Nursing and yet Weaning?

Most medical professional believe that you should start introducing cow's milk when your child is at least one year old. Some moms supplement with cow's milk during the weaning process and others prefer alternatives like formula or Pediasure. It boils down to individual taste. If your child is allergic to cow's milk, you may need to seek alternatives like almond or soy. Whichever you choose, ask your physician before proceeding and always watch for signs of allergy or intolerance. A rash, diarrhea, gas or noticeable fussiness may mean your child has an intolerance to cow's milk.

Since I'm not Producing As Much Milk As I Used to, Do I Water Down the Milk or Supplement? How Do I Know When I'm Giving Too Much or not Enough?

You don't need to water down your breast milk if you're trying to wean. Instead, you can simply substitute another nutritious drink (Pediasure, formula, cow's milk, or watered-down juice) to ensure your child is receiving the nutrition they need. These liquids will keep baby hydrated during the weaning process. If you choose to give your child watered-down juice, limit juice and use good dental hygiene to avoid cavities.

How Many Liquids Do I Need to Give My Baby When Weaning? How Do I Know If I'm Providing Enough?

Your baby's diapers will let you know if they're getting enough liquid. Their urine should not be dark yellow (this means dehydration), and their stools should be soft and easy to pass. If you see signs of dehydration, offer them something to drink (whether it's milk or water) in a sippy cup, or a cup with a straw if they're old enough to handle these. If not, put the liquid in a bottle and encourage frequent drinking. Also, always, always, always seek medical attention if you have any concerns about whether your baby is dehydrated.

What Should I Do When My Child Wants to Nurse During the Weaning Process?

One of the most common ways to handle this is to give a "replacement" for the breastmilk. For instance, if you're introducing cow's milk, you can give this to your baby instead of nursing (assuming they have no allergies) to breast milk. Another option is to distract your child with cuddles or a story instead. As long as they're not hungry, you may be able to supplement the nursing session.

How Much Milk Do Mothers Typically Produce During the Weaning Process?

Breast milk production is connected to hormones and typically a "supply and demand" system. In other words, the less your baby nurses, the less milk your body will produce. The weaning process needs to be done gradually though for this to happen without causing you pain or discomfort.

What Is Normal Milk Production for a Working Mother During the Weaning Process?

The amount of milk produced depends on how much your baby is nursing and whether you're pumping. If you are in the process of weaning, it is perfectly normal to start out pumping 2 or 3 times a day. As you go through the weaning process, you want to reduce these sessions gradually. For instance, you may go from 3 sessions down to 2 then 1. Keep in mind that the more you pump, the more you're telling your body to produce milk.

What Are Some Recipes or Food Ideas During the Weaning Process?

Fruits such as bananas, pears and avocados are excellent first foods for baby-led weaning, as well as steamed vegetables such as sweet potatoes and carrots. Some other choices are small pieces of peaches or cut-up cucumbers. Focus on softer items such as pasta, small peach slices, and soft steamed veggies, and then work up to firmer foods like apple pieces and cheese slices. If you choose veggies, you may want to use a crinkle-style cutter to make them easier to hold. In practicality, be open to trying food items that the rest of the family enjoy.

What Are Some Natural Ways to Avoid Mastitis or Engorgement When Weaning?

If you find that your breasts feel full and uncomfortable at times when you would have been nursing, you can use a breast pump or manually extract a very small amount of milk. Just enough to relieve the pain. This process helps your body adjust milk production to the level required by your baby. You can also try pumping to alleviate pain and discomfort. If you find that you're engorged, you can use cold compresses and cabbage leaves. Both help with swelling and pain. The purple variety of cabbage works best. Tylenol or Motrin can also be used as long as there are no contraindications.

Wean that Kid!

Importance of a Weaning Support Team

A weaning support team can make a world of difference for a weaning child, mother, and even father. Weaning a child can be a difficult time, particularly for one who has developed a routine that feels comfortable and safe.

Older children who are weaned are often able to vocalize their needs and wants for support, affection, and understanding during the weaning process. Many children express their unhappiness with the weaning process. This can be frustrating for a mother who is working diligently to support her toddler through the weaning process.

Weaning isn't only difficult for toddlers, however. Mothers often find that once they begin the weaning process, the emotional toll is harder than expected. Breastfeeding helps both child and mom establish a comfortable and relaxing routine. Weaning represents a shift in that routine and can sometimes result in mixed emotions, regret, sadness, and confusion. Even gradual weaning can present challenges for mothers and their babies.

Some mothers aren't certain that they will be able to let go of their breastfeeding relationship at the time they feel is right to wean. Some normal feelings that moms experience include sensations of loss and guilt. These are normal and are not an indication that anything is wrong with the weaning process. Time is usually necessary for both mom and child to adapt to the weaning process.

A weaning support team can help reduce the stress and tension that is sometimes associated with weaning. The primary member of a mom's support team may be her partner. A husband will be able to provide additional love, support, and affection and cuddle time for both child and mom when the time to wean arrives. Just as a young one sometimes needs additional affection, so too does a mother who is weaning her child.

A partner can also help both mother and child adjust their routine so they get used to interacting in ways other than breastfeeding. Most men will welcome the opportunity to be an active participant in their wives' and children's lives once again.

Many mothers turn to their mothers and other family members for support and understanding during the weaning process. Your mom and other female family members will be able to provide you with insight regarding their weaning challenges and emotional feelings. They can help distract you and reassure you that weaning is a natural part of your child's development. They can also help distract your child and take part in activities designed to distract babies from breastfeeding.

When weaning, a mom can also find support among other mothers who are nursing and weaning. Consider joining a local support group for breastfeeding mothers or mothers of toddlers. Engage your child in new activities by joining a playgroup. You will find comfort and reassurance in the stories, struggles, and successes of other mothers who have gone through similar trials and tribulations. You'll likely also pick up on a variety of useful tips that will help you during your weaning process.

A good weaning support team will provide you with the following:

- Encouragement

- Support and understanding

- Love and affection

- Help caring for your weaning child

- Ideas for distracting your youngster

- A shoulder to cry on

- Someone to talk to in times of stress

- Reassurance that you are making decisions that are best for you and your child

If you are isolated or don't have the opportunity to get out and join a community support group, there are hundreds of online support communities and chat groups related to breastfeeding and weaning. You can chat with mothers around the world about their breastfeeding, weaning, and childcare experiences. Feel free to solicit advice and share your stories with thousands of moms who truly understand where you are coming from.

By sharing your thoughts, feelings, worries, and concerns, you'll discover that you are more relaxed and better prepared to provide your child with the emotional support and love needed during the weaning process.

Conclusion

The decision to wean is one that requires careful consideration and a good, long look at your present relationship with your child. Try to screen out the voices of the people around you and focus instead on what your body and your mind are telling you to do. Keep in mind that you will feel better equipped for the challenges ahead if you do your research on the subject, write down your plan of action, stay positive and confident, and reach out to the ones you love for help and support. Be honest with yourself about your expectations and goals, and remember change is always a little difficult at the outset. Nevertheless, change is also a wonderful part of life. Remember that the weaning process marks the beginning of an exciting new chapter for you and your growing child.

Wean that Kid!

Weaning Resources

1. La Leche League International

http://www.lalecheleague.org/

La Leche League was founded to give information and encouragement, mainly through personal help, to all mothers who want to breastfeed their babies. LLL believes that breastfeeding, with its many important physical and psychological advantages, is best for baby and mother, and is the ideal way to initiate good parent-child relationships.

2. Jane's Breastfeeding Resources

http://www.breastfeeding.co.uk/

Jane's Breastfeeding Resources, at *www.breastfeeding.co.uk*, is an excellent gateway to breastfeeding information.

3. Breastfeeding Basics

http://www.breastfeedingbasics.com/

This site covers *Everything You Always Wanted to Know About Breastfeeding, But Didn't Know Who to Ask*. Offers knowledge, information, and resources (accessories) to help nursing mothers.

4. Nursing Mothers Alliance

http://www.nursingmothersalliance.org

Nursing Mothers Alliance is a volunteer, non-profit organization that serves many areas in the western suburbs of Philadelphia. The Alliance offers non-medical telephone counseling by trained lay counselors who have breastfed at least one baby for six months or more.

5. Lactation Education Consultants

http://www.lactationeducationconsultants.com

Provides prospective lactation consultants and other health professionals with programs related to lactation and breastfeeding information that is practical, current, and evidence-based.

6. Bright Future Lactation Resource Centre Ltd.

http://www.bflrc.com

Provides clinical and professional education, staff assessment, and training, consultation with hospitals and agencies, networking and referrals, resource analysis, and research for policy development.

7. Lactation Connection

http://www.lactationconnection.com

Provides tried and true breastfeeding and baby products that meet and exceed customers' standards, as well as cutting-edge technology in breast expression. Lactation Connection uses only manufacturers that have the breastfeeding mother at heart. Shop with confidence!

8. Eaglevideo.com

http://www.eaglevideo.com

Features an award-winning educational video on breastfeeding benefits that comes just in time with the most updated medical information! "The Benefits of Breastfeeding" offers the facts mothers-to-be need to know in order to make an *informed* decision on one of the most important health choices for their newborn.

9. Breastfeeding Your Baby (BabyCenter.com)

http://www.babycenter.com/breastfeeding

23 "Ask the Expert" articles, life stories, and polls centered on breastfeeding including weaning, readiness and extended feeding.

10. LaborofLove.com Articles Index

http://www.thelaboroflove.com

A wealth of information on breastfeeding, weaning and difficulties.

11. Breastfeeding USA

http://www.breastfeedingUSA.org

Empowering you with mother to mother support. Includes articles to help as well as a list of breastfeeding counselors throughout the United States.

12. Just Breastfeeding.com

http://www.justbreastfeeding.com/

Informative blog run by an Internationally Board Certified Lactation Consultant, ICCE Certified Childbirth Educator, Certified Labor Doula, and author. Most importantly, Danielle is a mother who as been through the birth experience twice.

13. Luna Lactation and Wellness

http://www.lunalactation.com

Luna Lactation & Wellness is committed to providing personalized, comprehensive support for all phases of lactation and beyond. We view lactation as a holistic process and respect each family's unique health care beliefs. We strive to provide nurturing, clinical care so that each family can define their own feeding and wellness goals.

14. Kelly Mom

http://kellymom.com

The KellyMom.com website consists of evidence-based informational articles and links to further information on breastfeeding and parenting topics.

15. BreastfeedingOnline.com

http://www.breastfeedingonline.com

This site is run by Cindy Curtis, RNC, Certified Lactation Consultant since 1993 and a Registered Nurse since 1996 and contains articles of interest and great resources to take to your doctor's.

16. Breastfeeding at Women's Health.gov

http://www.womenshealth.gov/breastfeeding/

A federal government website managed by the Office on Women's Health through the U.S. Department of Health and Human Services. Includes downloadable PDFs with information and helpful information whether you want to nurse for two weeks or two plus years.

17. Breastfeeding Resources at Centers for Disease Control

http://www.cdc.gov/breastfeeding/

The CDC is committed to increasing breastfeeding rates throughout the United States and to promoting and supporting optimal breastfeeding practices toward the ultimate goal of improving the public's health. An incredible amount of resources is available here.

18. ZipMilk

http://www.zipmilk.org

A complete database of breastfeeding resources broken down by zip codes, includes information on providers, consultants and resources for moms.

19. WicWorks Breastfeeding Resources

http://wicworks.nal.usda.gov/breastfeeding

This site is run by the US Department of Agriculture and provides links to agencies that support breastfeeding as well as articles, printouts and other online resources.

20. Health e-Learning.com

https://www.health-e-learning.com/

Resources offered by the International Institute of Human Lactation, Inc.

Tools to Make the Weaning Process Easier

Determining Whether You're Ready to Wean Your Kid

Now it is time to see if you're ready to wean your child. To do so, please be completely honest with yourself. Take a moment to think about the following questions and how they affect you and your child, and then write down your sincere answers. Once you do that, figure out if you're ready to wean your kid.

1.   How do you feel about your child's nursing sessions? Do you find the contact enjoyable, burdensome, a nurturing experience, or an interference with your personal freedom?

_____

_____

_____

_____

_____

2.   Does your child still enjoy nursing? If so, are there any other things that your child also enjoys?

_____

_____

_____

_____

_____

3.   Are you tired of other people complaining about your child nursing, or do you become stressed when someone asks, "Is your child weaned yet?"

_____

_____

_____

_____

_____

4.   Do you feel extended nursing provides the same health benefits to both older and younger children?

_____

_____

_____

_____

_____

5.   Is breastfeeding the only way to soothe your child? If so, can you think of other ways that you can soothe your child?

_____

_____

_____

_____

_____

Breastfeeding Weaning Affirmations

My baby knows that I love her and she will get all of the nourishment she needs from his food.

The bond that I have developed with my baby will not go away; it will change and grow into a beautiful new bond, like a butterfly coming out of a cocoon.

My body is open to this next stage of my child's development and I am ready for this process.

My partner is ready to be more actively involved in the nourishment of our child. This is my gift to both of them.

Weaning is a natural part of my child's growth and development. We are both ready for this next step.

Gradually weaning my baby is what's best for both of us. We can ease into this in a natural rhythm.

My child is ready for this. This transition will be a positive, beautiful transition.

I have a new found sense of freedom in this next stage of our life. I will embrace all of the opportunities for love and laughter that are placed before me.

Rollercoasters of emotion are a natural part of this process. I will move through them gracefully and know that laughing and exercising are natural remedies to help me find an emotional balance.

I will give myself extra love and care during this time of changes in my life.

I understand that I am feeling vulnerable now and I will make sure to seek out things that make me smile.

Wean that Kid!

Table I. The Weaning Progress Tracker

	Number of Occurrences	Average Duration	Comments (feelings, obstacles, changes, etc.)
Week 1			
Day 1			
Day 2			
Day 3			
Day 4			
Day 5			
Day 6			
Day 7			

	Number of Occurrences	Average Duration	Comments (feelings, obstacles, changes, etc.)
Week 2			
Day 1			
Day 2			
Day 3			
Day 4			
Day 5			
Day 6			
Day 7			
Week 3			
Day 1			

	Number of Occurrences	Average Duration	Comments (feelings, obstacles, changes, etc.)
Day 2			
Day 3			
Day 4			
Day 5			
Day 6			
Day 7			
Week 4			
Day 1			
Day 2			
Day 3			
Day 4			

	Number of Occurrences	Average Duration	Comments (feelings, obstacles, changes, etc.)
Day 5			
Day 6			
Day 7			
Week 5			
Day 1			
Day 2			
Day 3			
Day 4			
Day 5			
Day 6			
Day 7			

	Number of Occurrences	Average Duration	Comments (feelings, obstacles, changes, etc.)
Week 6			
Day 1			
Day 2			
Day 3			
Day 4			
Day 5			
Day 6			
Day 7			
Week 7			
Day 1			

	Number of Occurrences	Average Duration	Comments (feelings, obstacles, changes, etc.)
Day 2			
Day 3			
Day 4			
Day 5			
Day 6			
Day 7			
Week 8			
Day 1			
Day 2			
Day 3			
Day 4			

	Number of Occurrences	Average Duration	Comments (feelings, obstacles, changes, etc.)
Day 5			
Day 6			
Day 7			
Week 9			
Day 1			
Day 2			
Day 3			
Day 4			
Day 5			
Day 6			
Day 7			

	Number of Occurrences	Average Duration	Comments (feelings, obstacles, changes, etc.)
Week 10			
Day 1			
Day 2			
Day 3			
Day 4			
Day 5			
Day 6			
Day 7			
Week 11			
Day 1			

	Number of Occurrences	Average Duration	Comments (feelings, obstacles, changes, etc.)
Day 2			
Day 3			
Day 4			
Day 5			
Day 6			
Day 7			
Week 12			
Day 1			
Day 2			
Day 3			
Day 4			

	Number of Occurrences	Average Duration	Comments (feelings, obstacles, changes, etc.)
Day 5			
Day 6			
Day 7			
Week 13			
Day 1			
Day 2			
Day 3			
Day 4			
Day 5			
Day 6			
Day 7			

	Number of Occurrences	Average Duration	Comments (feelings, obstacles, changes, etc.)
Week 14			
Day 1			
Day 2			
Day 3			
Day 4			
Day 5			
Day 6			
Day 7			
Week 15			
Day 1			

	Number of Occurrences	Average Duration	Comments (feelings, obstacles, changes, etc.)
Day 2			
Day 3			
Day 4			
Day 5			
Day 6			
Day 7			

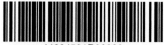

Made in the USA
San Bernardino, CA
26 January 2017